HOLD FAST

AIGBEFO D. EHIHI

HOLD FAST

A STORY OF HOPE & INTERVENTION

Aishific Press

Hold Fast: A Story of Hope & Intervention

Copyright © 2024 by Aigbefo D. Ehihi. All rights reserved.

No part of this publication may be reproduced in any form, or by any means, electronic or mechanical, including photocopying, recording, or any information browsing, storage, or retrieval system, without permission in writing from the publisher.

Unless otherwise indicated, all the characters in this book are fictitious. Any resemblance to actual persons, living or dead, is purely coincidental.

Paperback ISBN: 979-8-8693-3453-4
E-book ISBN: 979-8-8693-3454-1
Library of Congress Control Number: 2024909803

Aishific Press
www.aishificpress.com

Aishific Press titles may be purchased in bulk for educational, business, fundraising, or sales promotional use. For more information, please email books@aishificpress.com

Printed in the United States
First Printing, 2024

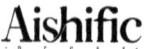

CONTENTS

Introduction
3

1 — The Storm
9

2 — A Cry in the Night
21

3 — The Morning Light
30

4 — The Binding Thread
40

5 — The Harvest Of Hands
49

CONTENTS

6 — The Echoes Of Fellowship
60

7 — The Northern Bound
71

8 — When Resilience Is Tested
80

9 — Bridging Home And Duty
89

10 — Shadows In The Fall
99

11 — Foundations Of Faith And Family
108

12 — In The Footsteps Of Faith
117

13 — Legacy Of Light
126

14 — The Lifeline of Connection
132

CONTENTS

15 — Echoes Of Change
137

16 — Epilogue
143

DEDICATION

To my beloved wife, Olubunmi P. Ehihi, whose relentless support and inspiration have profoundly shaped my journey.

AKNOWLEDGEMENT

———————

My heartfelt gratitude goes out to my beloved wife, fellow chaplains, and all those who have selflessly invested in me. Your unwavering commitment to supporting me has fueled my determination and inspired me to reach others with uplifting messages.

INTRODUCTION

A theatrical event unveiled a previously concealed crisis in the serene village of Fort Reachie, where the ocean shares its secrets with those who care to listen. This dramatic event lays bare what will shake the faith of the citizens. "Hold Fast: A Story of Hope & Intervention" is a captivating story of battle, redemption, and the unyielding power of faith. It is a narrative that aims to shed light on the often-overlooked grinds of individuals, especially our patriotic service members, facing mental health challenges. Here, where every suffering is felt profoundly, and every joy resonates loudly, the story of one man fighting against despair unfurls a narrative that echoes the journey many leaders encounter in silence.

COL James Aish (not his real name), a distinguished and highly decorated army officer, finds himself at the center of this flurry. He grapples with his internal struggles as a man with unwavering discipline and profound ethical beliefs. In addition to his external challenges, his inner conflict is often a personal battle against his thoughts. In his pursuit of saving someone else, James is poised to either find his own freedom or be overwhelmed by the depths of his unvoiced sorrow.

Just as the waves crash against the shores of Fort Reachie, that is how the storms of our soul attack the barriers we erect to shield us from these assaults. This work of fiction explores the true meaning of holding fast in the face of the crushing cyclones of life, with mental health challenges at its core. It testifies to the resilience of the human spirit, even in the most challenging circumstances.

It also underscores the transformative power of faith and the support of a community, which play a crucial role in James's journey. In the quietude of a restless night, I realized that our stories about our most challenging times carry a light powerful enough to guide others through their struggles or darkest moments. Just as Christians reflect on David's well-known words in Psalms 23:4, "Even though I walk through the valley of the shadow of death, I will fear no evil," "Hold Fast: A Story of Hope & Intervention" was born from a similar moment. It is inspired by the less popular story in Acts 16:28, where Paul prevented a desperate guard from taking his own life. These passages form the background of our story and serve as a beacon of hope that we are not alone, even in our darkest moments in the valley.

This book is an elaborate masterpiece of interwoven stories. It is deeply rooted in the real-world challenges of mental health and the issues surrounding suicide. Through the lives of Col. Aish and young Michael, we will explore the intricacies of mental illness and the stigmas that often silence those who are suffering. We will also delve into the transformative power of faith and community in addressing these painful realities. Besides being a theme in this story, the power of faith and community inspires all readers. Inspiration like this turns the tides of hopelessness into redemption.

As a Christian author, I aim to shed light on the often-overlooked crises many face, especially our patriotic service members. By featuring an army officer as the main character who offers help and experiences suffering, I hope to break down prejudices and encourage a more understanding and supportive approach to mental health. The story demonstrates the healing and transformative influence of faith and community, providing a ray of hope in our most difficult times.

'Hold Fast: A Story of Hope & Intervention' will introduce you to characters whose ordeals echo the raw human emotion we all share. These characters find themselves in situations that demand bravery and must submit to a higher calling of faith, love, and duty. This book is a message to all who are fearfully tottering on the edge of life, those who bear the world's weight on their shoulders, and those who believe they must face it alone: Hold fast, for hope is closer than you realize.

Hold fast, for intervention is traveling your way. The struggles depicted in this narrative, whether they be the chaos of war or the battle against mental health challenges, are not unique. They are universal. Moreover, through this universality, we find strength and support in each other. It reminds us that we are all in this together, and our shared experiences can promote understanding while comforting us in the process.

I desire that you will find relief in knowing that your struggles do not go unnoticed and that there is always a hand reaching out in the community of faith, especially in your darkest moment, ready to pull you back into the light. Even when you may not see the inviting hand at first, if you can hang in there and look through the slitting light piercing through the darkness, you will receive the help you need. You are not alone in your struggles, and there is always hope.

In his letter to the Romans, Paul encourages them to rejoice when they encounter trials or challenges in life, as these experiences help us navigate life and build endurance. He explains that enduring difficult situations helps to develop our character. This character formation strengthens our hope, which will not lead to disappointment. I pray this story inspires you to show empathy and understanding to those facing mental health challenges and to be a source of support in their lives, fostering a sense of compassion in the audience.

CHAPTER 1

THE STORM

COL James Aish stands in the quiet solitude of his study. His study room wall is lined with bookshelves filled with military histories and classic literature. Entering this study room immediately reveals James's mind as one seeking understanding in war and peace in chaos. Today, his uniform hangs ready on a stand, and the medals and ribbons fastened to the chest portray a narrative of valor and honorable service to our nation and beyond. Nevertheless, the uniform's pristine condition belies the turmoil in the man wearing it.

James's hands are steady as they have been trained to be, but his mind is a blizzard of memories. It must be incredibly tough to carry such heavy memories. Looking out the window as the storm gathers over his hometown, it is as if his outside turmoil reflects his inner turmoil. The chaos of war seems to have left a lasting impact on him, reminding him of the sudden shifts and the loss of his comrades. It is heartbreaking to imagine the pain he must be feeling.

Today, James faces a different kind of battle. It is not with an enemy combatant but with the invisible adversary of PTSD, along with the heavy burden of Moral Injury that haunts him during quiet moments. The heavy air before the storm feels like the building pressure before a flashback, a suffocating weight that he is all too familiar with. On days like this, when the weather changes and the wind whispers of impending fury, his mind tends to wander down difficult paths.

Despite all these happenings, James has an important speech to prepare for Veterans' Day. He anticipated the speech to inspire and remind others of the sacrifices and honor of service. As he turns away from the window and sits at his desk, a sturdy oak piece that has borne the weight of countless decisions, he carries the weight of his experiences.

At this time, James repurposes this sturdy oak desk to deliberate something other than war strategies. It is now a platform to convey the experiences of soldiers and foster understanding among those directly involved in combat, those welcoming them back, and those observing military life from a distance. His writing serves as a healing process, with each word becoming a deliberate step forward. He emphasizes courage as the ability to confront fear regardless of the situation.

He talks about the unity that soldiers, irrespective of their background, rank, or position, discover through their shared experiences and the unspoken gesture of respect that can convey more than a thousand words. James understands that his message must transcend mere words as he provides wisdom and guidance to those navigating their challenges.

The distant rumble of thunder gently ushers in the first drops of rain, creating a soothing, rhythmic patter against the windowpane that seems to synchronize with his typing. Each drop resonates with James's intense focus on his task, as if he is still a soldier serving and fighting but now on a battlefield of the mind, memory, and emotion. As he pauses, takes a deep breath, and finds a strange sense of solace in the storm's approach, it is evident that he embraced it as a personal challenge.

In the face of the raging storm that devastated Fort Reachie, James, a resilient professional soldier, continues to find solace in his writing. With each word, he seeks to first heal his wounded spirit. With each sentence, he takes a step closer to finding inner peace. And with each statement, James offers comfort to his reshaped emotions. This Veterans'

Day, James will be honored for his remarkable service as a retired Colonel. He will also stand as a symbol of encouragement for all individuals struggling with the invisible wounds of war and for those affected by it.

The rain intensifies, shrouding Fort Reachie as James hammers out his speech. Then, a sudden, sharp crack of lightning slices through the sky, briefly illuminating his room with stark, white light. In that split second of brilliance, James catches sight of something unexpected. It was a figure standing at his gate, soaked to the bone, a uniform clinging to a frame that carries burdens similar to his own. This is no ghost from his past, no apparition from the battlegrounds that haunt him. It is Sergeant Daniel Marsh, a young man who served under James's command. This man should not be standing in the gale, but instead, somewhere safe, somewhere dry.

Without a second thought, James rises from his desk, his Veterans' Day speech forgotten, as he rushes to the door. He throws it open to the raging elements, the wind howling a protest as he strides toward the figure. "Daniel!" he calls out, his voice barely rising above the storm's clamor. The young soldier looks up, his eyes reflecting the storm's chaos and something more, a turmoil that James recognizes all too well. "What are you doing here, son?" James inquires, his tone a mix of concern and reprimand as he ushers the drenched soldier inside.

"I... I didn't know where else to go, sir," Daniel admits, his voice breaking over the words. "It is the storm, sir. It brings it all back... and my family, they don't understand." Inside, the warmth of the house embraces Daniel, a contrast to the cold barrage outside. James guides him to the living room, urging him into a chair. He moves efficiently, fetching towels and a blanket, and James's role as a protector instinctively takes over.

As Daniel dries off, James sees the younger man's hands shake, the tremors more intense than the chill of the rain. Sitting across from Daniel, James leans in, his eyes fixed on Daniel's. "You did the right thing coming here," he says with assurance. You are not alone in this. The storm—it's not just in the sky; it is in us. But we face it like we face everything else. We face it together."

James then decides to do something he has not done before. He reaches for the speech on his desk, the words he crafted for others, and begins to read aloud. As he reads, what fills the room is the tale of bravery, hidden wounds, and standing together against the unseen enemy. As the words continue to fill the room, the storm outside seems to lessen, with the thunder receding into a distant rumble. This was probably because the tale of bravery sent the storm's rage into a distance as James read louder and louder.

However, the most remarkable change occurs in Daniel. His shoulders, once hunched like a man carrying the world's weight, begin to ease as he listens. The words of his former commander, not speaking from a podium or in front of the formation but from across the room, become a beacon in his storm. "What we have gone through marks us, but it does not define us," James concludes, setting the pages down. "And tomorrow, when I give this speech, I want you to be there, Daniel. Not just as a spectator but as a part of it. This village needs to see the faces of the brave as much as they hear their stories."

Daniel nods, a silent covenant forming between the two warriors. In this unexpected moment, on the eve of Veterans' Day, they find an unexpected camaraderie, not amid war, but in the shared battle against the relentless storm of Moral Injury and PTSD. James's speech, once just an arrangement of words, now takes on a new life and purpose. It becomes a vessel for healing, a balm for the wounded heart, and profoundly attests to the unspoken bond between those who have served and suffered.

As the first light of dawn peeks through the clouds, breaking the hold of the storm, James and Daniel sit in quiet contemplation, both aware that the road to recovery is long and fraught with challenges. However, in this shared space, they find strength, understanding that while the storm may rage, it can also cleanse. And in its wake, it leaves behind a fresh canvas upon which new beginnings can be sketched.

In the silence that follows the storm's retreat, SGT Daniel Marsh looks towards COL James Aish, seeing not just his former commander but a kindred spirit. This guidepost ushered him through the squall to a haven of understanding and empathy. He finds relief in the fact that the haunting echoes of the battlefield have an antithesis in the fellowship of those who shared those domains. The room's quietness starkly contrasts the dissonance that reigned moments before. There, surrounded by remnants of James's military past and the sanctity of his home, the two soldiers are simply men, each bearing scars seen and unseen, each seeking peace in the aftermath of the storm.

James stands, feeling a renewed sense of purpose stirring within him. With gentle authority, he suggests, "Let's make some coffee. It will be a long day, and we'll need all the strength we can muster." As they move to the kitchen, the early light reveals the aftermath of the night's fury—a scattering of debris, branches torn from trees, a community shaken but still standing. It mirrors their internal landscapes, a physical manifestation of their turmoil. Pouring two cups of coffee, James offers one to Daniel, who accepts it with a nod of thanks. They sip in silence, the warmth of the brew a small comfort against the lingering chill. Then, James speaks his words, cutting through the quiet.

"You know, Daniel, what we experienced last night, what we feel after every storm, is a reminder that we can withstand much more than we often believe. And it is also a reminder that we need to reach out, to find those anchors in our lives that keep us grounded." Daniel listens, the truth of James's words resonating within him. He has been afloat for too long, caught in the swells of his private storm. Nevertheless, in the presence of someone who understands, he begins to see a path forward.

James places a hand on Daniel's shoulder, a silent message of camaraderie. "We will rebuild not just the town but ourselves. And we will do it together, as a community. Your family and the people out there may not understand what we have been through, but they will stand with us. We just have to let them in." With the daylight strengthening, the town of Fort Reachie begins to stir, its people emerging to assess and repair the damage left in the storm's wake. The sight is an emotional reminder to both men that healing is not a solitary effort but a communal one.

As they finish their coffee, James turns to Daniel with a determined look. "Let's start the clean-up outside. It is time to set things right." Together, they step out into the street alongside their neighbors; they work tirelessly to clear the storm's remnants, finding comfort in the shared effort. With each branch cleared and every word of support exchanged, they felt the weight of the storm's shadow lifted, bringing renewed hope to all. Today, they are more than veterans; they are active community members bonded by shared purpose, battle, and renewed hope.

Furthermore, when COL James Aish stands to speak later that day, his words will carry the weight of experience and the promise of a future where no internal or external storm can shake the foundations of Fort Reachie. His words resonated with the depth of knowledge, experience, and promise of a future where Fort Reachie stood firm, upheld by its resilient people and unbreakable bonds forged through service.

CHAPTER 2

A CRY IN THE NIGHT

Late one evening, James receives a distressing call from Linda, whose teenage son, Michael, has vanished after leaving a troubling note. Recalling the scripture from Acts 16:28, "Do yourself no harm, for we are all here," James immediately sets out in the storm to find Michael, driven by a deep sense of duty and compassion. The lingering clouds from the earlier storm deepen the darkness of the night. Streetlights cast a dim, uncertain glow on the wet pavement, while the occasional flicker of distant lightning provides a silent countenance to the evening's urgency. James, gripping his phone tightly after the jarring ring that shattered the quiet of his home, moves with swift purpose.

Linda's voice, filled with concern and tinged with urgency, reverberates in James's mind. She had characterized the note as unclear yet unsettling; a few hastily scrawled lines expressing disillusionment and a longing to break free. James empathizes with the youth's struggles, particularly in a town weighed down by expectations and buffeted by coastal winds. Speedily, he buttons up his jacket against the lingering chill of the storm and strides out into the night. His strides are long and determined, the soles of his boots meeting the wet earth in a steady rhythm.

James recognizes the places where the young people of Fort Reachie seek comfort during tough times. It is the cliffs overlooking the cataclysmic sea where the land seems to understand the deep yearning for freedom and the consolation of the untamed. The rugged and imposing cliffs have a remarkable way of showcasing the might and beauty of nature, a poignant contradiction to the turmoil within Michael's heart.

As he approaches the cliffs, his sharp eyes catch the faintest movement and a shadow against the restless backdrop of the ocean. Michael stands recklessly close to the edge, a lone human outline barely noticeable against the dark expanse of the water. James's heart clenches as a reaction honed from years in combat, where every second can mean the difference between a life saved and a life lost. "Michael!" James's voice carries on the wind, firm yet imbued with the warmth of concern. The boy does not turn, but he stiffens, aware now that he is no longer alone in the abyss.

Carefully, James approaches, each step measured, his every sense attuned to the young man's posture, to the tension that speaks of a soul in turmoil. "I will not pretend to know exactly what you are going through, Michael,"

James begins, stopping a safe distance away. "But I do understand the feeling of being at the edge, of looking into the deep and wondering what is looking back." His words, filled with empathy and shared experience, create a bridge of understanding between them.

The rolling waves crash against the cliffs, a soundtrack to their precarious moment. Michael's voice, when he speaks, is barely louder than the whisper of the sea spray. "It is like being caught in a crosscurrent," he confesses, his words carried to James on the wind. "You fight and fight, and it still pulls you under." James nods, acknowledging the raw truth in the metaphor. "I have been there, in the grips of a current that wants to take everything. The key is to remember that the crosscurrent is not the whole ocean. There is calm, too. There is hope. And there are people who are ready to swim out and bring you back ashore."

It is a standoff with the darkest parts of the human psyche; James faces the same courage he bore in war but with a different kind of strength. His is the strength of vulnerability, shared experience, reaching out, and holding on. Slowly, Michael turns, his eyes meeting James's, the connection between them a lifeline in the swelling darkness. Together, they walk back from the edge, away from the siren call of the abyss, moving toward the promise of dawn and the community that awaits, ready to uphold them both.

The night's cry for help does not go unanswered, and as they leave the cliffs behind, a new understanding is forged between James and Michael and within the heart of Fort Reachie. This community stands vigil, even through the darkest nights. The power of community support, like a bonfire in the night, guides them back to safety and hope. As they walk back, the world around them is quiet. It mirrors the occasional stirrings of wildlife and the distant echo of waves. Their footsteps are the only sign of life on the deserted path. James senses the young man's hesitance and reluctance to leave the solitude of the cliffs for the reality waiting for him at home. He knows this walk is not just a physical journey back to town but a passage from despair to hope, from isolation to community.

"You know, Michael," James initiates the conversation, breaking the silence between them. When I was overseas, we used the term 'watch your six.' It means looking out for each other and protecting one another. It is something we could use more of back here. Michael listens, his gaze on the ground, his mind processing the words. James continues, drawing from the well of his own experiences, "The battles we fight do not always look like we expect. Sometimes, the enemy is in the mirror or the thoughts that keep us awake at night." He stops and turns to face Michael. His features are etched with sincerity in the moonlight breaking through the dissipating clouds: "We all need someone to watch our six, Michael. We all need someone to lean on in times like this.

No one is meant to face the dark alone." It is a simple statement, yet it carries the weight of undeniable truth. Michael's eyes finally lift to meet James's. There is a dawning realization in them, a spark of something dimmed by his struggles. It is a plain recognition of his worth in the eyes of another. James reaches into his pocket, pulling out a challenge coin emblazoned with his unit's insignia. He places it in Michael's hand, closing the young man's fingers around it. "This coin means you are never alone. It means someone's got your back that you are part of something bigger than your battles."

Cool to the touch, the coin grounds Michael in the present, connecting him to a significant moment of the forged connection. James speaks of the soldiers who carry these coins, their belief in never leaving a comrade behind, the strength in unity, and the courage to admit vulnerability. Their conversation turns to stories of soldiers who faced their internal storms and emerged stronger, of communities that rallied to support those who had borne the weight of freedom on their shoulders. These tales from James do not glorify or diminish the struggles.

James uses these tales to illuminate the

path to healing while inspiring Michael with real-life examples of resilience and recovery. By the time they reach the edge of town, the first hints of dawn are painting the sky with strokes of orange and pink. A new day is on the horizon, and the promise of a fresh start comes with it. James's offer to Michael is simple: join him later that day at a community gathering and have a chance to see and be part of the support network in Fort Reachie. Michael agrees, the challenge coin a tangible reminder in his pocket of the lifeline extended to him.

Moreover, as they part ways at the town's threshold, with James assuring him they will meet again soon, Michael walks home with a new perspective. He has learned that strength does not always roar; sometimes, it is the quiet voice at the end of the day whispering, 'I will try again tomorrow.' Thus, James successfully imparted the lesson to Michael and everyone who heard of that night. It is a lesson of the power of connection, the strength in community, and the enduring spirit of hope that watches over the village of Fort Reachie, even through the darkest storms and their lowest valley.

CHAPTER 3

THE MORNING LIGHT

A beautiful and gentle morning in Fort Reachie brought with it the gentle kiss of sunlight, brushing away the remnants of night's shadow. The town, quaint with its cobblestone streets and historic storefronts, stirred to life as the scent of freshly baked bread and the sound of opening shutters drifted in the air. COL James Aish was already up despite the early hour, the night events having charged him with a restless energy.

He sipped his black and strong coffee on the porch of his white-paneled house, watching as his neighbors emerged to greet the day. Each friendly wave and smile served as a reminder of the town's unspoken creed: Here, people did not just look out for one another; they were a part of each other's lives, a community bound by a shared sense of belonging.

James's heart swelled with a renewed commitment to his community after his encounter with Michael and Sergeant Daniel Marsh's unexpected visit. Today was not just another day; it was the day he had been quietly preparing for, the day to introduce the support program. His speech from the night before, now laden with deeper meaning, rested on the kitchen table, ready to be shared. As the town's clock tower chimed eight, James set off for the community center, a sturdy brick building that stood as a hub of local activity and a lighthouse for fellowship.

The center was already abuzz with the

preparations for the Veterans' Day commemoration, a tradition in Fort Reachie that drew out the town's residents and folks from neighboring areas. The flutter of flags and the arrangement of chairs created a sense of anticipation and unity. Amidst the flutter of flags and the arranging of chairs, James found Linda, Michael's mother, supervising a group of volunteers. Her face brightened upon seeing him, a mixture of relief and gratitude evident in her eyes. They exchanged a few words, her voice quivering as she thanked him for finding her son. James offered a comforting hand on her shoulder, assuring her that Michael was stronger than he knew.

As the hour drew near, the residents began to fill the seats. The young and old veterans came in a procession of pride and humility, their shared service creating an unspoken bond that transcended generations. Among them, James spotted Daniel, standing a bit apart, his eyes scanning the crowd until they landed on his former commander. A silent nod exchanged between them spoke volumes.

Then, there was Michael, looking out of place amongst the uniformed men and women yet bearing a similar look of searching, of needing to belong. James beckoned him over, introducing him to Daniel. The two exchanged tentative greetings, the beginning threads of a new support network forming. With the community gathered, James took the podium.

The sun, now high and radiant, cast a warm glow on the faces before him. He began to speak, his voice steady and sure. He spoke of service and sacrifice, of the battles fought in distant lands and those fought within the recesses of the heart. He also spoke of the invisible wounds of war, the wounds that bled into everyday life, leaving scars unseen but deeply felt. As he shared his vision for the support program, he invited the audience to join him in standing watch over those who had served, to be the keepers of each other's six.

He explained that The program would offer counseling, resources, and activities designed to bridge the gap between military and civilian life, heal, and fortify. James's words were met with applause, nods of understanding, and eyes glistening with the first tears of healing. However, it was his following invitation that drew a collective breath from the crowd. "I ask any among you who have felt the riptide to stand," James said, his gaze sweeping across the audience. Slowly, veterans rose from their seats, joined by civilians—mothers, fathers, children, and friends—each representing their battles with adversity.

In that moment, the room was filled with a palpable sense of shared experiences, a collective determination to overcome, and the transformative power of hope as they all stood together, united in their resilience. Michael, his heart pounding with a mix of anticipation and hope, rose to his feet. Beside him, Daniel stood taller, his posture a reflection of the strength he had found in this community. The sight of the standing crowd, a patchwork of Fort Reachie, was a powerful symbol of the resilience and unity inherent in the human spirit.

James's voice, filled with conviction, rang

out, "Today, we stand united, not just in remembrance, but in the commitment to heal, thrive and lift each other from the depths. Today, we are all keepers of the six." The event closed with renewed hope, and conversations budded among strangers and friends alike. They made plans as volunteers signed up. Michael and Daniel, drawn together by their shared experiences, discussed the program with a newfound eagerness to participate, a spark of optimism in their eyes. Clearly, the support program had already begun to make a difference, instilling a sense of belonging and hope in those who had felt lost and alone.

The unity and commitment of the community, as demonstrated in this event, was a beacon of inspiration for all. The impact of the support program was evident in the rekindled hope and sense of belonging it brought to Michael, Daniel, and the entire community. As the day waned and the crowd dispersed, James remained a moment longer, looking over the now-empty chairs, feeling the weight of what had been started. The Veterans' Day event sparked a movement in this small coastal village. It was one that promised to watch over its own with the same enthusiasm with which they had watched over others. In Fort Reachie, morning light had brought a new dawn of understanding, compassion, and hope. It is now a community united in the promise to hold fast, come what may.

In the quiet aftermath of the gathering, as the last of the attendees trickled away in small, intimate groups, the actual depth of the day's impact began to reveal itself. Upon picking up a fallen flag from the ground, James reflected on the symbol in his hand, the colors vibrant against the backdrop of a clear blue sky. The flag was more than a symbol of a nation; it represented the people within it, of their resilience and capacity to rise, time and time again, no matter the adversity faced.

A young boy, no more than ten, approached James, his eyes wide with the innocence and curiosity that children possess. "COL Aish," he began, his voice a hesitant whisper, "my daddy says you are a hero. Were you not scared when you were a soldier?" James knelt to the boy's level, his expression softening. "Being brave does not mean you are not scared," he explained gently. "It means you do what is right, even when scared. It is like standing up for a friend, even when you face a bully. It is doing the small good things, even when they seem hard." The boy digested this, and then his face brightened. "I can be brave too, then!"

"Yes, you can," James affirmed, a smile tugging at his lips. "Every day, we can all be brave in little ways. That's how we make the world better." James rose as the boy ran off, likely to share his new understanding of bravery. The brief interaction was a poignant reminder that the day's lessons extended beyond the adults and veterans; they touched even the youngest minds among them. Inspired, James decided to extend the community event with an impromptu lesson in civic responsibility for the children.

With the help of a few volunteers, they quickly organized a mini-parade for the children, where each could carry a small flag and march around the community center. It was a lesson in patriotism, sure, but also in community engagement and mutual support. As the children marched, laughter and chatter filling the air, James took the opportunity to instill a more passionate message. "Each flag you carry," he told them, "represents your part in our community. Like each of us, they are different but create something beautiful together."

The children, energized by their role in the day's events, asked questions and shared their dreams of who they wanted to become. Some spoke of military aspirations, while others shared simpler but no less critical ambitions. Some shared how they want to be teachers, doctors, or even to make the best pizza in Fort Reachie. James listened, realizing that this was another facet of his mission: to teach the next generation the values of courage, community service, and integrity. "Your dreams," he said to the gathering of eager faces, "are like these flags. You must hold them high, care for them, and never let them touch the ground, no matter what storms come."

The Veterans' Day event, which had begun as a solemn remembrance and a call to action for support and understanding, had grown into something more significant. It had become a multi-generational promise, a pledge from the people of Fort Reachie to uphold the values that defined their town and the very essence of what it meant to be part of a community. James felt a deep contentment as the sun dipped lower in the sky, casting long shadows on the playing children. Fort Reachie had shown that it was a place where the legacy of the past fortified the dreams of the future. Within that legacy, today's lessons would help mold the citizens of tomorrow.

CHAPTER 4

THE BINDING THREAD

In the quiet that followed the day's celebrations, Fort Reachie seemed to breathe a collective sigh of contentment. Nevertheless, for COL James Aish, the work was far from over. The seed of change had been planted, and he was keen to nurture it. At the heart of the town, the community center's lights still glowed, a watchtower for the evening's quieter work. Inside, James, alongside a dedicated team of volunteers, began mapping out the new support program earnestly. They started by identifying the community's needs and resources and then planned for regular counseling sessions, skill-building workshops, and community outreach events. They also drew charts, assigned roles, and created a calendar of events.

The program, named "The Binding Thread," symbolized the strength and connectivity of the community fabric. As they worked, James noticed Linda hovering near the doorway, her presence hesitant but purposeful. Approaching her, he saw the remix of hope and concern etched on her face. She held out a casserole dish, a peace offering to the busy volunteers. "James, I... I want to do more," Linda confessed after some small talk about the day. Her voice trembled with a mix of hope and fear. "After what you did for Michael, for all of us today, I feel like I need to be part of this change. I have seen the impact of your work, and I want to be a part of it."

Her words struck a chord with James. The

program needed champions, individuals willing to transform their gratitude into action. "We are honored to have you, Linda," he responded, his voice infused with sincerity. "Your perspective as a parent, your understanding of what it is like to almost lose someone to the shadows is priceless." Linda's inclusion brought a new dynamic to the team. She represented the families of those who struggled, the ones who watched from the sidelines, often feeling helpless. Her input was well received and actively sought after. Linda shared her experiences and suggestions, which helped shape family outreach initiatives and support systems that they later integrated into the program.

Daniel and Michael arrived as the night progressed, their earlier hesitance replaced by a cautious eagerness to contribute. They sat with James, Linda, and the other volunteers, sharing their insights into the struggles faced by returning veterans and troubled youth. Michael spoke up, his voice steady, "Maybe we could start a mentorship program where vets like Daniel can share their experiences and help kids like me feel less... adrift." Inspired by Michael's suggestion, Daniel added, "And maybe include some skills workshops. Sometimes, having a mission, feeling useful, can make all the difference."

Their ideas received enthusiastic approval, and "The Binding Thread" started to come to life. It was a triumphant moment, showcasing the power of teamwork. The program was becoming comprehensive, providing emotional support, practical skills, and engagement opportunities. James stood before the volunteer team as the meeting ended, his heart brimming with pride. "This," he said, motioning to the room filled with dedicated faces, "embodies the true spirit of 'watching our six.' We are creating something that goes beyond individual experiences and brings us all together."

The team disbanded for the night, each member carrying a spark ignited by the promise of the work ahead. James lingered longer, reviewing the notes and plans scattered across the tables. Those papers lay the framework for a future where no one in Fort Reachie would feel alone. It will be a village that will meet every struggle with adequate support and where the ties of the community will be the binding thread that holds them together. It was a vision of hope, a promise of a brighter future.

Under the quiet watch of the stars, the town of Fort Reachie slept, its residents unaware that within the humble walls of the community center, a new chapter had begun. It is a chapter where each person, each story, became part of a more extensive embroidery, rich with the colors of shared humanity and woven with the strength of collective resilience. Fort Reachie, a small village with a big heart, was home to a diverse community, each with their struggles and triumphs. 'The Binding Thread' responded to these challenges, a testament to the village's resilience and commitment to collective well-being.

In the serenity of the night, with the distant sound of the sea whispering through the community center's open windows, James was the last to leave. He turned off the lights, but before locking up, he paused. The silence spoke to him, as did the empty chairs and the plans scattered like fallen leaves on the tables. It was a profound moment of solitude, a time to reflect on the power of a single day to alter the course of many lives. Then, James made a quiet decision: he would begin a journal of "The Binding Thread." It would not be a mere record of events and dates but a chronicle of transformation, a collection of narratives that would one day tell how a town healed itself from within.

He started that very night. Under a lone lamp, with pen and paper borrowed from the community center's supply closet, he began to write. He wrote of the day's victories, the forming of new alliances, and the seeds of ideas that, if tended with care, would grow into sturdy oaks under which many could find shelter. "The Binding Thread," he wrote, "is not just a support program. It's a testament to our collective spirit.

It is proof that every act of kindness, every offer of support, and every shared burden can strengthen the weave of our community. Like threads crossing in a tapestry, we are stronger together than we ever could be apart." This journal would be a gift to the future, a lesson for those who might one day face their storms, and a reminder that no effort to help others is too small and no reach for help is too great. James kept writing over the following weeks as "The Binding Thread" took shape.

He described Linda's remarkable bravery in facing the challenges of loving someone who grapples with unseen inner struggles. He documented Daniel's progression from a place of doubt to becoming a solid source of support for others, and he portrayed Michael's transformation from the edge of hopelessness to a beacon of encouragement for his peers. These narratives were more than just stories; they were robust evidence of the program's ability to bring about profound change.

The journal became a tapestry, interwoven with the threads of personal growth and community triumph. Each entry was an inspiration, a lesson in the humble alchemy that turns individual experiences into collective wisdom. In one particular entry, James details a Saturday when the veterans and youth reunited to restore an old playground. They painted faded swing sets, repaired broken seesaws, and replaced the gravel with soft, safe sand. It was a metaphor not lost on those who worked shoulder to shoulder. These people were rebuilding a place for joy, just as they were rebuilding the joy within themselves.

On another page, he described how Michael had started a peer counseling group where young people could talk without judgment. It was a circle of trust that expanded with each session as more and more youths came, drawn by the power of shared experience and the promise of understanding. There was also the veterans' storytelling evening, where Daniel and others shared tales of their service. The tales comprise heroic moments, doubts, fears, and camaraderie. These stories stripped away the gloss of glory to reveal the true face of bravery. He portrayed this face of bravery as perseverance, vulnerability, and the willingness to continue serving, even in civilian life.

James's journal and "The Binding Thread" grew, each influencing the other, reflecting a community finding its way towards something resembling healing. He saw Fort Reachie progressing towards a future where no one would be left to weather their storms alone. As James continues the journal, the entries are not just records; they are lanterns, lighting the way for others to follow, proving that everyone can contribute to the community's strength.

This narrative would serve as a blueprint for other communities, a case study of compassion, and a chronicle of the unassuming heroism in caring for one another. In Fort Reachie, the days passed, but the thread remained, binding them all, a golden line of hope intertwined through the villagers' hearts. It glistened most brightly in the moments when it was needed most.

CHAPTER 5

THE HARVEST OF HANDS

Autumn arrived in Fort Reachie, clothing the town in vibrant hues of gold and crimson. The air was crisp, filled with the scent of burning leaves and the distant sound of the high school band practicing for the homecoming game. It was a harvest time for the farmers with their bountiful yields as it was also for "The Binding Thread," which was beginning to reap the fruits of its labor. COL James Aish, a dedicated pioneer of 'The Binding Thread, 'watched from his porch as children scurried by, their laughter a merry accompaniment to the rustling leaves.

His journal lay open on his lap, the pages now filled with numerous accounts of small victories and giant leaps toward healing. Nevertheless, today, he was not writing. Instead, he was more involved in observing and contemplating. He was eyeing the full circle of growth, the change of natural seasons, and the human heart. The village was bustling with excitement as the "Harvest of Hands" festival kicked off at the community center. This event was an excellent opportunity to showcase the fantastic work of "The Binding Thread" and raise funds for its programs.

The festival aimed to highlight the town's creativity and generosity, with local vendors offering a wide array of handmade crafts, delicious baked goods, and fresh harvest produce. It was a beautiful demonstration of the community's diverse talents and shared accomplishments, underscoring the power of unity and support. Linda, a dedicated member of 'The Binding Thread,' managed the registration booth gracefully, welcoming volunteers and visitors with a genuine warmth that brightened everyone's day. Her newfound confidence and clear communication skills were invaluable to the festival's success, and her caring nature made her a reassuring presence for many. Her exceptional organizational abilities played a pivotal role in ensuring the festival ran smoothly and efficiently.

In the vicinity, Daniel, Michael, and other veterans and youths hosted a booth highlighting collaborative community art projects. These projects aimed to capture the community's essence and its members' experiences. The canvases were filled with vibrant colors and powerful imagery, depicting stories of hardship, hope, and unity. Each piece revealed the artist's journey, an open letter of their path through darkness toward light. James mingled with the crowd, sharing handshakes and stories as the day progressed. He felt immense pride in witnessing the community's progress in fostering camaraderie and shared understanding. His attention was drawn to a quieter booth with a simple setup featuring a banner titled "Stories of Service."

Attendees were encouraged to sit and engage as veterans shared their stories. Each account was distinct, showcasing the range of experiences and the common thread of service. The focus was not on glorifying war but on understanding the challenges of service and the journey back to civilian life. It was a space for empathetic listening, mutual respect, and knowledge sharing. While the narratives were diverse, they all revolved around themes of sacrifice, resilience, and the ongoing need for support. The festival's "Circle of Thanks" event began as the late afternoon sun cast a warm glow.

Residents formed a large circle in the town square, each holding a piece of yarn. Starting with James, the yarn traversed from hand to hand, uniting the crowd physically and symbolically. Addressing the assembly, James spoke about the intention behind "The Binding Thread," expressing the aspiration that no one in the community should ever feel isolated in their struggles. He lifted the linked loop of yarn and conveyed that it represented collective hope and strength, a tangible symbol of the community's commitment to supporting one another.

During the "Circle of Thanks," the community shared a moment of reflection on the challenges and progress they have experienced over the years. They thought of bonds formed with neighbors and friends, sons and daughters, loved ones, and strangers who had become family through shared experiences and mutual support. As the festival wrapped up, James put his thoughts to paper. He described the day as a celebration of the land's bounty and the collective kindness and collaboration among people. He wrote "The Harvest of Hands" as a reminder that our acts of compassion yield a rich and supportive community."

The day drew to a close as the sun dipped

below the horizon, casting long shadows over the pages of his journal. These pages chronicled the story of Fort Reachie. It is evident that every community holds the potential for greatness, awaiting the right hands to cultivate it, the right hearts to nurture it, and the collective spirit to bring forth abundance.

James penned his final reflections for the day in the fading light as the townsfolk basked in a soft glow. Drawing inspiration from the biblical account in Acts 16:28, where Paul urgently told the jailer, "Do not harm yourself, for we are all here," James found resonance with the day's theme. Paul was not judgmental; he did not ask why and did not hesitate despite being a victim. He did not leave the jailer alone; he led the jailer away from self-harm, leaving a significant and eternal impact. The passage emphasized the importance of being present for one another, especially those facing challenges, regardless of how we may feel about them or how they treat us. It is a value that Fort Reachie exemplified in full measure.

James looked around at the dispersing

crowd and considered the strength from knowing others were there, a collective force against the tide of individual struggles. The "Harvest of Hands" festival was quite a celebration. It was also a declaration that echoed Paul's protective call. It said, "We are here, we are with you, and you are not alone." James observed a poignant scene in the softening light as the yarn from the "Circle of Thanks" was carefully collected and placed around the base of the community center's flagpole.

A young girl approached Daniel shyly, asking if she could hear his story of finding purpose. With gentle eyes, he knelt to meet her gaze and began to share. He shared heartfelt war stories, returning home, finding purpose, and communal integration. The girl listened, enthralled, then looked up at Daniel with understanding beyond her years. She showed great empathy, drawing parallels between Daniel's experience and the story of the jailer and Paul. "So you were like the jailer, hopeless, scared, and alone, and COL Aish was like Paul, telling you not to hurt yourself because help was there?" she asked.

Daniel smiled, surprised by her insight. "Yes, I suppose that's right," he affirmed. "And now you are like Paul for others, right?" Her question was innocent but profound. "Exactly," Daniel nodded. "Just like all of us can be. We can all look out for each other." The conversation continued, with the young girl asking more questions and Daniel sharing more of his experiences, fostering a deeper connection and understanding. It was a living illustration of the scripture, a modern-day reenactment of that ancient truth. The people of Fort Reachie were embodying the message that had echoed through the ages, standing as guardians for one another, ensuring that no one faced their darkest hours alone.

James included this exchange in his journal, capturing the essence of the interaction and its broader implications. "Tonight," he wrote, "a young child reminded us of the power we each hold to be a force of comfort and safety for one another. Like Paul in the cell, we are called to be the voice that calls out in the darkness, offers hope when all seems lost, and physically represents God's love, grace, and care." The day's celebration reaffirmed the villager's commitment to one another. Just as Paul had been there for the jailer, and the jailer had found new life and purpose through Paul's intervention, so had the people of Fort Reachie found new strength in their togetherness.

James closed the chapter with a prayer of thanks for the enduring spirit of community fostered in Fort Reachie. He prayed that the ties that bound each person to another would remain strong, even as seasons changed and years passed. He prayed that the lessons of this day would resonate in the hearts of all who participated, rippling out to touch even those who had yet to join their circle. "May we always remember the call of Acts 16:28," James wrote, his handwriting steady and sure, "and may we always respond with the same urgency, compassion, and dedication. Let us hold fast to the truth that our presence can be the lifeline someone desperately needs, and let us never hesitate to extend our hands, to share our stories, and to offer our support."

As he finished writing, James looked upon the flagpole, the yarn encircling it like a bandage healing a wound. It symbolized their collective commitment, a testament to their unity. Moreover, beneath the flag, waving gently in the evening breeze, the community of Fort Reachie stood represented, a patchwork of individuals united in purpose and love. With that, James closed his journal, the leather cover holding the stories of a town that had come together to heal, grow, and stand as a beacon of hope. It was a living document that he knew would continue to grow with each new challenge and victory they would face together.

Looking at how the "Harvest of Hands" festival thrived, James felt a deep sense of peace as the stars twinkled above, mirroring the lights slowly coming to life in the houses around the square. The voices of Fort Reachie whispered through the night, carrying with them the promise that no cry for help would go unanswered, for they were all there, each for the other, as their threads of hope continued.

CHAPTER 6

THE ECHOES OF FELLOWSHIP

The days in Fort Reachie grew shorter as winter approached, and the nights arrived earlier with a chill that whispered of the coming season. However, within the community center, a place that embraced them all, warmth pervaded from the hearth and the hearts and actions of those gathered within. The Binding Thread's embroidery had grown rich with the stories and lives of the villagers, each strand an inimitable part of the whole.

On a particularly frosty evening, as James made his way to the center for the monthly town hall meeting, he could not help but reflect on the vibrant transformation that had taken root. The streets, once quiet avenues for solitary walks and contemplative silence, now thrived with the chatter of neighbors and the cheerful, chaotic mixture of life lived in fellowship.

The hall was arranged in a circle, chairs facing inward, fostering a sense of belonging and unity. The walls were adorned with the colorful arrases of 'The Binding Thread,' each strand representing a unique story and life. The gathering was not just for sharing updates but also for reinforcing the bond that had become the very essence of the community. James took his seat among his fellow residents, each person there a living proof of the strength of their collective spirit.

The meeting commenced with a moving prayer led by Pastor Alinko, a deeply respected spiritual guide invited to offer his wisdom and support. His words resonated with a sense of healing as he invoked the presence and the grace of the Prince of Peace to accompany their collective endeavors. Pastor Alinko's message centered on the idea that their actions testified to their unwavering faith. He again drew inspiration from Acts 16, drawing parallels between Paul's declaration of safety and presence and the very essence of their shared purpose. He encouraged everyone to be fully present for each other, offering support and affirmation, irrespective of circumstances or personal feelings.

The floor was then opened for testimonies, a time for anyone to share their struggles and triumphs. An older gentleman, Mr. Phranklin, a veteran of life's many battles, stood first. He spoke of his loneliness after his wife passed away during one of his deployments and how The Binding Thread had become his family. His voice, thick with emotion, echoed in the hearts of all present.

Tears welled in many eyes, and a collective

sigh of empathy filled the room. "It is like that scripture we keep hearing about," Mr. Phranklin said, steadying himself on the back of a chair. Paul's call to the jailer was a call to eternal life. And you all have been that call for me. I thought my days of feeling were over, but you have shown me that there is a life yet to be lived, even for an old man like me."

Philomena, a young mother, gracefully rose from her seat, holding her daughter's delicate hand. Her daughter had come into the world six weeks earlier than expected, facing the challenges of being born prematurely. Philomena courageously shared her story of navigating the complexities of caring for a premature baby, as well as her experience with postpartum depression and the isolating feelings that often accompany it. "I felt trapped in my own home, in my mind," she confessed. "But Linda reached out. She became my Paul, reminding me I was not alone and was surrounded by a community that cared."

As the testimonials continued, James felt the threads of every story, every life, weaving a tapestry that depicted the full spectrum of human experience—sorrow and joy, despair and hope. It was a powerful reminder that their shared humanity was the most vital thread of all, evoking a deep sense of empathy and understanding.

The town hall meeting transitioned into a crucial planning session for the winter outreach initiative. Now rising to the challenge, Daniel proposed "Winter's Warmth," a program to ensure that no one in Fort Reachie would be without company or care during the coldest months. It would include meal deliveries, snow removal services, and regular wellness check-ins, particularly for the senior citizens and infirm. Each resident's input was valued and considered, emphasizing the importance of their contribution to the community.

Daniel's proposal sweetened James's heart to the point where he shared tears of joy. The initiative was met with resounding approval and a flood of volunteers. Teenagers paired with seniors, veterans with families, and new mothers with those whose children had long since grown. It was a project that would provide physical warmth and kindle the warmth of human connection in the face of winter's cold embrace.

As the meeting neared its end, with plans in place and hearts uplifted, James felt a deep sense of connection and compassion. It represented the enduring bond between individuals, reminiscent of the fellowship between Paul and the jailer. It emphasizes the importance of offering support not only in times of crisis or to those we like or know but also to everyone in the everyday moments of existence.

It stood as a testament to the solemn pledge to "Do not harm yourself, for we are all here" - a promise that resonated through every member of the community, acknowledging and honoring the unique contributions of each individual. 'The Binding Thread' symbolized their intertwined stories and lives, weaving a poignant tapestry of communal experiences and unwavering support.

James left the community center that night with a notebook under his arm, full of fresh entries for his journal. Each word he would write was a testament to the enduring spirit of Fort Reachie. This town had become a living example of the power of fellowship and the strength of a promise kept, even under the most ordinary of circumstances. James, too, had played a part in this transformation, his contributions a thread in the tapestry of Fort Reachie.

As the winter nights grew longer and the cold air settled more firmly over Fort Reachie, the community's spirit of mutual support became even more vital. Inspired by the proactive steps the town had taken, James decided to add a new feature to "The Binding Thread" initiative, a storytelling night called "Fireside Tales." This would be a monthly event where people from all walks of life could come together, sharing stories and experiences in the warmth of a crackling fire at the community center. The event aimed to provide entertainment and deepen the sense of community and understanding among its members.

The inaugural "Fireside Tales" evening took

place on a particularly chilly night. A generous fire illuminated the stone fireplace at the heart of the venue, creating a warm and inviting atmosphere. The air was filled with the delightful aroma of burning wood, and the crackling of the fire in the background set a tranquil tone. Chairs and cushions were thoughtfully arranged in a semi-circle around the fire, encouraging guests to settle in and relax.

Attendees were treated to a selection of hot cocoa and tea, accompanied by delectable homemade buttermilk cookies, shortbread, and chocolate bars generously provided by talented local bakers. The room buzzed with laughter and excitement as individuals from diverse backgrounds congregated to share their stories.

As the attendees arrived, they wrapped their scarves tighter against the chill, creating an anticipation-filled atmosphere. James kicked off the event by explaining its purpose: "In the spirit of our community's bond, we gather here to share our stories—not just of hardship but of hope, of the mundane and the miraculous. In each tale, we find the threads of our shared human experience woven into a collective narrative that strengthens us all."

The first to share was Clara, a middle-aged woman who had recently moved to Fort Reachie. She shared the story of her first winter in town, when an unexpected blizzard caught her unprepared, and how her neighbors came to her aid by shoveling her driveway and inviting her over for dinner when her power went out. "I learned that night that a mountain of snow was no match for the warmth of this community," Clara said, her eyes shining by the fire.

Next, a teenage boy named Dale shared a different kind of story. He spoke about his struggle with anxiety, particularly about speaking in public. "Standing here now, telling my story, is something I never thought I would be able to do," he admitted, his voice shaky but strong. "But I have learned from many of you that being scared is okay. It's okay to ask for help. And every time I do, I feel a little stronger." His honesty resonated with the audience, and he was met with encouraging nods and smiles from around the fire.

Throughout the evening, each story added a new layer to the community's understanding of itself as people shared their challenges, moments of unexpected joy, and simple pleasures. The retired teacher, Mr. Nolan, fondly recounted his coaching days in the little league, reminiscing how those summer days on the baseball field brought him as much joy as his time in the classroom. James also shared a personal story about a difficult time during his military career when he felt secluded and unsure about his future.

He highlighted the impact of a fellow soldier who reached out to him during that challenging period, teaching him the profound effect of simple acts of kindness. As the fire dwindled and the last of the cookies were savored, community members lingered, unwilling to leave the comforting warmth of the fire and the camaraderie. These "Fireside Tales" had woven new threads into Fort Reachie's fabric, emphasizing the values of courage, laughter, and empathy.

It was evident that these shared experiences were crucial to the town's preparations for the winter, much like stockpiling wood for the fire or storing food for the cold months. This initiative had evolved the community center into a communal living room where individuals of all ages were valued and felt heard. The stories shared that night resonated through the chilly air, warmed the body, and kindled the soul while underscoring the deep-rooted caring nature of the people of Fort Reachie.

CHAPTER 7

THE NORTHERN BOUND

The winter had firmly gripped Fort Reachie, ushering in an unexpected call for COL James Aish. The military recognized his invaluable experience and leadership and asked him to temporarily return to duty. This is not a call to combat. It was a call to mentor, advise, and validate field training exercises at an Alaskan training base.

It was a temporary job preparing and validating young soldiers for Arctic operations in the Pacific. Given the geopolitical tensions in colder regions, this was a crucial task. James felt conflicted. He had become deeply entrenched in the community at Fort Reachie, fostering 'The Binding Thread' and nurturing the community's fabric.

However, he understood the need for his skills and experience in preparing soldiers for harsh conditions and high-stakes situations. After much contemplation, consultation with Pastor Alinko, and discussion with community leaders, James made the difficult decision to accept the assignment. He knew it was another way to serve, even if it meant being far from home. The community recognized his sacrifice and held him in even higher regard for his selflessness.

Before his departure, the community organized a send-off at the same community center where many of his initiatives had taken root. The room was filled with those touched by James's efforts—from elderly veterans to young children like Eli, who had found his voice thanks to James's supportive environment. "Your leadership has prepared us well, James," Pastor Alinko said during the event. "You have taught us that service does not end with a uniform. It is a lifelong commitment to lifting others up. We will keep the home fires burning until you return."

James headed to Alaska, well-prepared with warm clothing and a strong determination. Upon reaching Alaska, he was immediately struck by the stunning beauty of the icy landscapes. His base was north of Fairbanks, an ideal location for intense training due to the extreme temperatures. His responsibilities included imparting vital survival skills for operating in such a harsh environment, a task he was well-equipped for due to his extensive experience. Additionally, he validated major exercises as the units geared up for upcoming Pacific operations.

James dedicated his days to teaching young soldiers essential skills for surviving in the Arctic, such as setting up shelters and navigating through snowstorms. At night, he reflected on his experiences and kept up with news from Fort Reachie. During a challenging training session, James observed the soldiers' coordinated efforts. He saw evidence of his positive influence on their determination and skills. He knew that his guidance had prepared them well for their assignments and fostered personal growth and resilience in each of them.

Amidst the harsh and rigorous regimental training in the remote Alaskan wilderness, Captain James managed to carve out a precious moment to foster an ardent sense of camaraderie among his fellow soldiers. Against the backdrop of snow-capped mountains and under the starlit sky, James introduced his rendition of "Fireside Tales" to the base, inviting everyone to gather around a crackling bonfire.

As the flames danced and cast flickering shadows, he encouraged his comrades to share heartfelt stories from their homes, the reasons that propelled them into service, and their aspirations for the future. This simple yet profound event served as a unifying force, reigniting the troops' spirits and strengthening their bond. It reminded each soldier that they were part of a larger narrative, with every individual playing a vital role in the collective mission.

As Christmas approached, the sense of isolation seemed to intensify against the breathtaking backdrop of the Alaskan winter. However, the base's chaplain, Benaiah, orchestrated a heartwarming celebration, adorning the space with a modestly decorated tree. The exchange of handcrafted gifts, each carrying a piece of home, provided a much-needed touch of comfort and familiarity amid the icy wilderness. The soldiers' shared sense of belonging and unity was palpable, defying the harsh isolation that enveloped them.

James's time in Alaska became a testament to his unyielding dedication to service, whether within the warmth of Fort Reachie or the unforgiving cold of the Arctic. He emerged as a bridge between these contrasting worlds, and each experience instilled a profound appreciation for the enduring value of community and resilience. His journey underscored the unchanging and essential principles of leadership, empathy, and fellowship, which remained unwavering and unyielding, much like the resolute winter ground beneath the mesmerizing dance of the northern lights.

As James's assignment in Alaska pressed on, he immersed himself in the grueling physical demands and unique challenges of Arctic training. Amid these trials, a newfound opportunity for learning emerged—not only for the young soldiers under his command but for James himself. He learned that the survival techniques applicable in the Arctic could double as potent metaphors for personal and emotional resilience, concepts he was enthusiastic to instill in his trainees and share with his community back home.

One bone-chilling morning, James rallied the troops for a specialized training session dedicated to physical survival and mental fortitude. His chaplain, chief training Noncommissioned Officer (NCO), and James co-led this session. Chaplain Benaiah introduced the "Iceberg Principle," a term he coined to illustrate the significance of acknowledging the unseen facets of any challenge, similar to the vast portion of an iceberg concealed beneath the water's surface.

"Just as we must anticipate and respect the hidden dangers of an iceberg in these waters," Chaplain Benaiah explained, gesturing towards a large chart with an iceberg illustration, "we must also be aware of the internal struggles we face, the stress, fear, loneliness that are not immediately visible to others." SGT Dion, the training NCO, set up an exercise where each soldier was tasked with building an emergency shelter, a standard training operation.

However, James added a twist this time: each soldier had to do it while sharing something personal about themselves with their team, an unseen challenge or thought they felt was necessary. This vulnerability exercise was designed to build trust and show that each person's unseen burdens were as critical to acknowledge and address as the physical tasks. The soldiers' personal growth and their progress in understanding and supporting each other was a source of pride for James and the entire community.

As the soldiers worked, the air filled with the sounds of crunching snow and candid conversations. Some shared worries about their families, others about personal fears of not measuring up, internal crises, and silent struggles, and some spoke of past failures they could not seem to shake. The exercise proved profound, tightening bonds among the soldiers and reinforcing the lesson that understanding and cooperation extend beyond physical aid. They also require emotional and mental health support.

Inspired by the success of this lesson, James decided to relay this experience to Fort Reachie by organizing a similar event remotely. He set up a video call during one of the community center's gatherings, where he shared his chaplain's insights on the Iceberg Principle and how it had helped his soldiers in Alaska.

This initiative, the 'Beneath the Surface' community group, was a testament to the unity and belonging that James had fostered in the community, even from a distance.

Back in Fort Reachie, community members listened intently, many nodding in agreement and understanding. They began discussing how this principle applied to their lives, especially in dealing with unseen personal challenges. The discussion led to a new community group focused on mental health awareness. This initiative mirrored James's team's emotional vulnerability exercise with his soldiers.

This initiative quickly became integral to The Binding Thread, providing resources and regular meetings where community members could share their unseen struggles in a supportive environment. It was named "Beneath the Surface," a nod to the Iceberg Principle and a reminder of the importance of looking beyond what is immediately visible to truly support each other.

CHAPTER 8

WHEN RESILIENCE IS TESTED

The stark beauty of Alaska's winter landscape had been a silent witness to many training exercises, but none were as dire as what unfolded under COL James Aish's command. During a routine navigation drill designed to test the mettle and preparedness of young soldiers against the unforgiving Arctic conditions, tragedy struck.

A Light Medium Tactical Vehicle (LMTV) skidded on a patch of black ice, rolling over into a snow-packed embankment. The accident was severe. Two soldiers, young men recently out of basic training, lost their lives, and several others sustained injuries. The incident sent shockwaves through the unit, shaking the moral and emotional foundations of the soldiers who looked to James for leadership.

Deeply affected by the accident, James grappled with his leadership responsibilities. It was a moment that tested his professional and personal resilience as he faced the loss within his command in a training environment. The immediate hours following the accident were crucial. James's leadership team coordinated the emergency response, ensuring the injured received prompt medical care and that the families of the deceased were notified with respect and sensitivity.

After managing the immediate crisis, James turned his attention to the well-being of his unit. He recognized that the physical injuries, while pressing, were not the only wounds inflicted by the accident. The moral injury – the guilt, the grief, the shaken confidence – needed to be addressed if the unit was to recover and move forward.

In the days that followed, James organized debriefing sessions. He brought in military chaplains and counselors who had experience in crisis intervention. CH Benaiah conducted Traumatic Emergency Management (TEM) sessions. CH Benaiah held these sessions in the base's communal spaces, where the chaplain encouraged open dialogue and personal sharing. James spoke first, setting a tone of vulnerability and openness. "I know we are all feeling the weight of what happened," James addressed his unit, his voice steady but tinged with emotion.

"We have lost part of our family, and many of us are asking why—why this happened, what could have been done differently. It is normal to feel this way. It's human. But it's also our responsibility to learn, grow, and support each other through this. We owe it to those we have lost and those injured to look out for one another."

James implemented a buddy system, pairing soldiers together to ensure that no one was left to cope alone. He increased the frequency of mental health check-ins and introduced more informal gatherings where the soldiers could connect, share their feelings, and build back their sense of team cohesion without the formal structure of military drills. Understanding the power of ritual in healing, James's leadership organized a memorial service.

It was a simple yet profound ceremony, held at dawn with the breathtaking backdrop of Alaska's snow-covered peaks. Each soldier had the opportunity to say a few words, share memories of their fallen comrades, or stand in solidarity as they watched two lanterns float into the early morning sky. Through these actions, James demonstrated a fundamental military principle—that leadership is not just about directing others in tasks but guiding them through their experiences' complexities, especially in times of crisis. His leadership approach not only helped stabilize the unit. It also fostered a more profound sense of unity and mutual support among the soldiers.

As winter continued to grip the landscape, the unit began to find its footing again. Their resilience during this trying time was a testament to their bonds' strength and leadership quality. For James, the incident was a sad reminder of the weight of command and the profound capacity for recovery and growth that can arise from adversity. As the unit navigated the aftermath of the tragedy, James recognized the importance of continuing education and preparedness in physical maneuvers and emotional and psychological readiness.

To deepen this aspect of training, he introduced a new module called "Resilience Tactics," a program designed to integrate psychological resilience with physical training.

James collaborated with psychologists and military trainers to develop a curriculum that included stress management techniques, mindfulness practices, and scenarios designed to strengthen decision-making under pressure.

This training was not typical in military programs, but James believed fostering mental agility was as critical as physical preparedness. One of the most innovative aspects of "Resilience Tactics" was the introduction of simulation exercises that replicated physical challenges and emotional and moral dilemmas.

Soldiers were placed in high-stress environments where they had to make quick decisions involving tactical and ethical considerations. After each simulation, the unit would gather to debrief, discussing the tactics and the emotional responses triggered by the scenarios. These debriefings were guided by chaplains and mental health professionals who helped the soldiers articulate their feelings and thoughts about the decisions they had made.

This process encouraged deeper self-awareness and provided soldiers with real-time strategies to manage emotional stress. It also reinforced that acknowledging and discussing emotional reactions was not a sign of weakness but a strategy for strength. As the training progressed, the soldiers exhibited greater confidence in their physical tasks and ability to handle emotional and moral complexity. This growth was particularly evident during a field exercise designed to test their resilience. The soldiers were unexpectedly confronted with a simulated ethical dilemma involving civilian interactions. The choices were morally ambiguous and required careful consideration of immediate and long-term impacts.

The soldiers embraced the challenging exercise with maturity and thoughtfulness, reflecting their excellent training. During the debrief, many expressed feeling better prepared to handle similar situations in the future, acknowledging the complexities of real-world operations. This innovative approach began to draw attention from higher up in the military command.

Impressed by the reports of increased cohesion and resilience within the unit, other units expressed interest in adopting the "Resilience Tactics" program. These units invited James to present the results at a military leadership conference, where he shared insights and strategies, emphasizing the critical link between mental resilience and effective military operations.

The successful program highlighted a significant shift in military training methods, emphasizing the value of emotional intelligence and psychological fortitude. For James, the journey from the tragic incident to the creation and success of this program served as a powerful testament to proactive leadership and the importance of addressing all aspects of soldier readiness, both visible and invisible.

James concluded his time at the base as the winter deepened and the Northern Lights painted the Alaskan sky. He bid the soldiers farewell with a memorable evening of Fireside Tales, recounting their training and shared experiences. As James prepared to depart Alaska and return to Fort Reachie, he left an indelible impression on the soldiers he trained and contributed to a broader transformation in military training methodologies.

His efforts will ensure that the legacy of those lost in the accident lives on through the enhanced preparedness and resilience of numerous soldiers in the future. Returning to Fort Reachie, enriched by his time in Alaska, James brings back new survival skills and a deeper understanding of human resilience and the strength of community. He is poised to continue integrating these lessons into the fabric of his hometown.

CHAPTER 9

BRIDGING HOME AND DUTY

As the Alaskan winter thawed into spring, COL James Aish prepared for his return to Fort Reachie. At this time, his heart was heavy with mixed emotions. The 'Resilience Tactics' program, with its significant decrease in PTSD cases and other mental health issues and the increase in community cohesion, arguably impacted his leadership journey. It brought him a deep sense of professional fulfillment and marked significant personal growth as he grappled with the weight of the responsibilities that command bore. His journey was more than just professional. It was a personal journey marked by growth and resilience.

James's flight home was a long contemplation of his time in Alaska. He contemplated the lessons learned, and the resilience fostered within his troops and himself. He was returning not just as a leader who had expanded his experience in the harsh terrains of the Arctic but as a community leader whose vision had broadened far beyond the military aspects of leadership. He could not help but recall when he, too, participated in a community resilience workshop and how that experience had shaped his understanding of leadership and community development.

Upon his return, Fort Reachie greeted him with the warmth of a well-anticipated spring. The town had not been idle in his absence. The Binding Thread initiative had taken his ideas and run with them, weaving new programs and support systems that had strengthened the community fabric. James was eager to reconnect with this work and see how his contributions from afar had taken root at home.

The community center hosted a welcome-back gathering, where James shared stories from his time in Alaska. The villagers listened intently as he described the challenges of Arctic training, the tragic accident, and the subsequent triumphs in building resilience. His narrative was more of a bridge connecting his world in the military with the community efforts in Fort Reachie.

The 'Resilience Tactics' program inspired James to propose a new local initiative: a community resilience workshop series. The series would be open to all residents and offer training in first aid, crisis management, psychological first aid, and community leadership. The workshops were designed to empower individuals, equipping them with the skills to support each other in times of personal or collective crisis and to inspire them to take an active role in their community's development. The community leaders enthusiastically approved the proposal.

Sarah, a local teacher and a town council member, stepped forward to help lead the initiative. "James's experiences remind us that every member of our community has a role in our collective safety and well-being," she said during the meeting. These workshops will help us all become better prepared and more connected, emphasizing the crucial role of each individual in the community's success.

As spring progressed to summer, the community resilience workshops became a focal point of life in Fort Reachie. People from diverse backgrounds came together in a display of shared commitment. Teenagers partnered with elders, business owners collaborated with schoolteachers, and veterans joined forces with civilians. The sessions effectively enhanced skills and strengthened interpersonal bonds, creating a feeling of togetherness and common goals. One session, in particular, led by James, made a significant impact. "Building Emotional

Resilience in Difficult Times" helped participants acknowledge their inner strengths and learn how to utilize them for personal well-being and community assistance, showcasing the practical value of the workshops.

Reflecting on the past months and contemplating my continuous work in Fort Reachie, I am reminded of the impactful large-scale simulation of a town-wide emergency response we coordinated over the summer. This served as an exceptional opportunity to apply our training and exhibit Fort Reachie's heightened resilience. Witnessing the town swiftly mobilize, with each unit adeptly and calmly performing their roles, filled me with pride.

It became evident how seamlessly my roles as a military officer and community leader had intertwined. Each experience has enriched the other and laid the foundation for a comprehensive leadership approach practical in both civilian and military life. Fort Reachie now stands as a community-driven and resilience-focused leadership model. I eagerly anticipate our future progress. I am enthusiastic about the prospect of further inspiring other communities with our transformative journey said James.

As the summer waned and the flourishing community drill faded into a warm memory of collective achievement, James observed a growing curiosity among the villagers about the broader implications of their training. The community's newfound confidence in crisis management sparked discussions on utilizing these skills beyond mere preparedness. The aim is to transform the skills into proactive community development and leadership tools.

Inspired by this momentum, their community leader, Elder Crawford, proposed the next phase of the community's evolution: a leadership development program called "LeadReach." This initiative aimed to nurture emerging leaders within Fort Reachie by providing them with mentorship opportunities, advanced crisis management training, and projects addressing real-world community issues.

The program started with a series of workshops facilitated by James alongside other local leaders and guest speakers from various professional backgrounds. These sessions covered ethical decision-making, effective communication, and strategic planning. However, James was allowed to introduce an innovative twist to the training. Each participant was required to identify a community issue and design a project to handle it. The results were profoundly inspiring.

One group of participants, led by a young woman named Ellie, who had shown natural leadership during the summer drill, tackled the issue of food insecurity in Fort Reachie. They developed a plan to expand the community garden, partnering with local farmers and businesses to provide fresh produce to residents in need. Their project addressed a crucial issue that strengthened the town's self-sufficiency in the long run.

Another group focused on youth engagement, creating a series of workshops and activities that connected younger residents with skilled mentors in various trades and professions. These kept teens engaged and out of trouble while equipping them with practical skills and potential job opportunities. The program quickly gained popularity and was set to become a staple in the community's educational offerings.

James took a step back in this phase of the community's development as these projects unfolded, allowing the new leaders to take the reins and offering guidance only when necessary. This approach helped foster a sense of ownership and accountability among the participants, reinforcing that leadership was not about wielding power but empowering others.

The LeadReach program culminated in a community showcase, where each group presented their projects and impacts on Fort Reachie. The event was well-attended, with residents eager to learn about the initiatives that their neighbors and friends had developed. The energy in the room was palpable, a mix of pride, excitement, and a collective sense of accomplishment.

Reflecting on the journey from the initial resilience training to the flourishing of

LeadReach, James realized the profound truth of leadership: it is most effective when it catalyzes others to realize their potential. By creating an environment where leadership skills could be practiced and honed in service to the community, James witnessed the cultivation of a new generation of leaders who would continue to drive Fort Reachie forward, instilling a sense of hope and optimism for the community's future.

As he penned his thoughts in his journal that night, James noted, "True leadership is like gardening. It's not just about planting seeds but nurturing them, watching them grow, and sometimes stepping back to let the new blossoms soak in the sun. Today, I saw a garden full of vibrant leaders ready to nurture their community, and I am reminded that our work is never just about the crises we face but the opportunities we create from them."

This chapter of Fort Reachie's story was just one of many. Still, it was clear that the community had transformed into a dynamic, self-sustaining ecosystem of leadership and innovation under James's stewardship. As autumn returned, painting the town in shades of gold and amber, James felt confident that the seeds of resilience planted during his leadership would continue to grow, evolve, and sustain Fort Reachie for many years.

CHAPTER 10

SHADOWS IN THE FALL

COL James Aish, a community pillar, watched as the leaves in Fort Reachie turned from gold to the deep, rich hues of autumn. The town, basking in the comfort of routine and the satisfaction of recent successes, was about to face an unexpected challenge. This challenge, brewing quietly beneath the surface of calm, would test the town's resilience in ways James had not anticipated.

The first hint of trouble came subtly, through minor disruptions that initially seemed like mere inconveniences. A series of small thefts occurred throughout the town—nothing major, but enough to stir whispers and unease among the residents. Items disappeared from backyards and porches—a bicycle here, garden tools there. These thefts, unsettling the community that had always prided itself on its trust and openness, were a blow to the very fabric of their unity.

James, ever vigilant, took note of the community's growing concerns. He discussed the incidents with the local sheriff, who had also observed an unusual pattern in these petty crimes. They seemed random, but their increasing frequency suggested something more than mere happenstance. During one of their strategy meetings, the sheriff received a call that a local store's security camera had caught a fleeting image of a suspect. The footage was grainy, and the figure was hooded, making identification difficult.

The mystery deepened as reports of similar thefts came from neighboring towns. A regional pattern emerged, indicating a more organized group of perpetrators rather than isolated incidents. This revelation brought a chill to the community, reminiscent of the icy winds soon to herald winter. James, recognizing the potential for fear to undermine all the community's work to build trust and resilience, decided to act.

He organized a town meeting to inform the community about what was happening and rally them around a response plan. The meeting was packed, the town hall buzzing with the low murmur of concerned citizens. Standing before his fellow residents, James spoke with calm authority. "We've faced challenges before," he began, his voice steady and reassuring. "And we have become stronger every time because we faced them together. This is no different. We will increase our vigilance, but not at the cost of our trust in each other.

We will set up neighborhood watches, support our local law enforcement, and keep our community informed every step of the way." The town's response was a unified nod of agreement. Committees were formed on the spot, schedules drawn up, and volunteers stepped forward to lead the watches. The atmosphere turned from worry to determined action as James's plan to safeguard the community took shape.

However, just as the meeting was about to adjourn, a young boy, Timmy, tugged at James's sleeve. He whispered something in James's ear that made him stiffen. Timmy claimed to have seen the suspect near the old mill on the outskirts of town—the mill that had been abandoned for decades. He spoke of strange noises and lights late at night. James thanked Timmy and promised to investigate, a thread of unease winding through his thoughts. The old mill was isolated, surrounded by dense woods—a perfect hideout. James stood at the back of the hall as the townspeople dispersed, his mind racing, a plan forming to safeguard their community.

The challenge had seemed straightforward, but Timmy's words hinted at a more profound mystery, perhaps more dangerous than simple thefts. As he set out to visit the old mill, the fading light casting long shadows across the town, James felt the weight of the unknown pressing down upon him. The quiet of the fall was about to be broken, and what lay in the shadows might shake the foundations of Fort Reachieh. James decided not to waste any time.

That evening, under the cloak of twilight, he set off towards the old mill, his instincts as both a soldier and a community leader guiding him. He understood the importance of addressing potential threats swiftly but cautiously, knowing well that fear and suspicion could undermine the fabric of trust and cooperation he had worked so hard to weave into the community. As he approached the mill, the crunch of dry leaves underfoot seemed unnaturally loud in the quiet of the night. The mill loomed ahead, its silhouette a dark blot against the fading light. James moved with purpose yet carefully, his senses sharpened by years of training.

Reaching the perimeter of the old building, James paused to survey the area. The mill, abandoned for years, had once been the heart of local industry but now stood as a forlorn monument to the past. The windows were boarded up, and the door hung loosely on its hinges. As he circled the building, his flashlight's beam caught something unusual—a fresh set of footprints in the soft earth leading towards the back of the mill.

Following the tracks, James discovered a poorly secured window that seemed to have been used recently. The realization that someone had indeed been using the mill was alarming. He noted every detail, aware that this clandestine activity could be the source of the recent disturbances in Fort Reachie. James carefully entered through the window, deciding it was crucial to gather more information before alerting the community or confronting whoever was inside.

Inside, the air was musty, filled with the scent of old wood and disuse. His light flickered across walls lined with graffiti, old machinery draped in cobwebs, and scattered debris. The far corner of the mill drew his attention. He saw a makeshift living area with blankets, food wrappers, and a small, battery-operated lantern.

As he inspected this setup, it became evident that this was more than a hideout for a thief. This was a refuge for someone in desperate circumstances. The realization softened James's initial vigilance into a renewed sense of purpose. Here was a person, or persons, possibly needing help rather than condemnation. This discovery marked a turning point, a moment of hope and empathy amid uncertainty. James's approach shifted.

He knew that Fort Reachie, with all its community spirit and resources, could support whoever sought refuge in this forgotten place. This was a moment to extend the community's

Reach and demonstrate that their resilience and unity could be inclusive, providing security, support, and rehabilitation.

The next day, James organized a discreet return to the mill with a small group of trusted community leaders and a social worker. They found two teenagers—a brother and sister—who had run away from a turbulent situation at home in a neighboring town. Scared and without a place to go, they found the old mill and made it their shelter.

The community leaders of Fort Reachie embraced the chance to aid the siblings, arranging for them to receive proper care and mediating a resolution with their families. The incident became a powerful testament to the values James had always championed: understanding, compassion, and community support.

Reflecting on these events in the next town meeting, James used the story to reinforce a critical message: "Every challenge we face is an opportunity to strengthen the bonds that hold us together. We must always look beyond the surface, seek understanding, and extend

HOLD FAST

our hand. Today, our community is not just safer but kinder and more connected.

Let us continue to protect and uplift one another, to build not just a town but a home for all." While initially a source of concern, the mill incident galvanized the whole of Fort Reachie, teaching valuable lessons in empathy, proactive kindness, and the true meaning of community. This lesson would resonate through Fort Reachie even to future generations.

CHAPTER 11

FOUNDATIONS OF FAITH AND FAMILY

As Fort Reachie's vibrant leaves turned into stark, wintry silhouettes, COL James Aish reflected more deeply on the core pillars that have upheld him through adversity and achievement. His unwavering faith in God and unwavering support from his family have been instrumental in sustaining him. Following recent events at the old mill and strengthening community ties, James felt a renewed appreciation for the personal foundations that anchored him. His relationship with God had always been a guiding light. God has always provided him and his family comfort during challenging times while magnifying moments of joy.

In the quiet mornings before the rest of the town awoke, James found reassurance in his Bible; its worn pages turned to passages that reminded him of resilience, providence, and God's love. One such morning, as dawn broke with a crimson glow casting through his window, James sat at his kitchen table with a cup of coffee and his Bible open to the Book of Joshua. "Have I not commanded you? Be strong and courageous. Do not be afraid; do not be discouraged, for the Lord your God will be with you wherever you go" (Joshua 1:9). This verse resonated deeply, echoing the journey he had undertaken, both in Fort Reachie and beyond.

James credited this unwavering faith for his leadership strength and commitment to service. Yet, he often mused that faith alone was not the entirety of his fortress. His family was equally foundational. His wife, Elizabeth, had been his steadfast partner through every deployment and every community challenge. Her wisdom, patience, and unwavering support had been his anchor in the most tumultuous seas. Elizabeth, ever perceptive, noticed James's contemplative mood one evening. Sitting beside him by the fireplace, she took his hand, her presence a silent invitation to share his thoughts. James spoke of the mill incident, the children they had helped, and how each challenge in Fort Reachie had brought the community closer.

He expressed how these experiences had underscored the importance of solid personal foundations. "You and the kids are my compass," James confessed, gently caressing Elizabeth's hand. "Knowing that you are there and believe in me makes all the difference. Our faith and family keep me grounded, help me serve better, and lead with compassion."

Elizabeth smiled, understanding the depths of his sentiment.

"We are in this together, always. Our faith, our love, our commitment—it is what makes us strong. It allows us to reach out and help others build their strong foundations." Encouraged and inspired by their conversation, this time, Elizabeth invested in a new community project involving families and fostering faith and familial bonds within Fort Reachie. They envisioned a "Family Faith Nights" series at the community center, where families could come together for an evening of fellowship, share meals, discuss scripture, and support one another in their spiritual journeys.

The success of the first Family Faith Night was a testament to the power of community and faith. Families gathered, sharing not just meals but also their stories and prayers. Elizabeth led the discussion on the importance of personal foundations, sharing her family's experiences and encouraging others to reflect on what kept them anchored. As children played and parents exchanged stories and prayers, a beautiful tapestry of shared values and mutual support was woven, a testament to the success of James's family initiative.

For James, watching the community come together in faith and fellowship reaffirmed his commitment to serving and leading with integrity. As winter deepened and the nights grew longer, the light of faith and the warmth of family continued to guide and inspire Fort Reachie, ensuring that no matter what challenges lay ahead, they would face them together, with God and each other as their surest guides.

As the Family Faith Nights became a cornerstone of the community's spiritual and social calendar, James observed an emerging dynamic that inspired him to take the initiative even further. He noticed that the adults were not the only ones benefiting from these gatherings; the children were forming connections and eager to participate in more than playtime, instilling a sense of hope and reassurance in the community's future.

Seizing upon this observation, James

proposed the addition of a Youth Mentorship Program to run parallel with the Family Faith Nights. This program would focus on teaching children and teenagers values like leadership, responsibility, and community service, all framed within the context of their faith. The idea was to foster a sense of agency in the younger community members, empowering them to think about how they could contribute positively to the world around them and inspiring them to become the future leaders and pillars of Fort Reachie.

With Elizabeth's help, who had a background in education, and the support of the local schoolteachers and church leaders, a curriculum that included practical life skills and spiritual teachings emerged. Each session began with a group discussion led by a rotating roster of mentors from various walks of life—local business owners, teachers, veterans, and even visiting guests outside Fort Reachie. These mentors shared personal stories of challenges and triumphs, linking their experiences back to the values and teachings of their faith.

One particularly impactful session was led by a local craftsman, Mr. Jacobs, who taught the kids woodworking skills. While they built birdhouses, Mr. Jacobs paralleled the careful crafting of these homes to building one's character. "Each nail, each piece of wood has its place, just as each trait and each act of kindness builds the shelter of your character," he explained. This hands-on approach kept the children engaged and helped them visualize and understand the discussed abstract concepts.

The kids, guided by their mentors, would also undertake a monthly community project. These projects ranged from organizing food drives for families in need to spending time with older adults in local nursing homes. This allowed them to put their faith into action while teaching them the importance of empathy and giving back. The positive feedback from parents was overwhelming. They reported seeing marked improvements in their children's attitudes and behaviors. Kids who once shied away from taking the initiative now lead community projects. Teenagers who struggled with direction were finding purpose in service and mentorship, building their self-esteem and moral foundations.

These transformations inspired James to document and share these stories in a monthly newsletter distributed within and beyond Fort Reachie. Each edition featured stories of the children's projects, their impacts, and reflections from the kids and their families. This newsletter soon garnered attention from neighboring towns, inspiring similar programs elsewhere and creating a network of communities engaged in youth mentorship based on faith and service.

As the seasons changed, with each new project and each Family Faith Night, the seeds James had planted continued to flourish. The initiative started to bind the community through shared values and support. However, it grew into a powerful movement that nurtured the next generation of leaders. James often reflected on this growth, proud and humbled by the role he had played. He knew that long after his time, the lessons of compassion, leadership, and faith sown today would blossom and sustain the community of Fort Reachie, echoing his deepest beliefs: that service is about planting trees under whose shade you do not plan to sit.

CHAPTER 12

IN THE FOOTSTEPS OF FAITH

As a dedicated leader of the Youth Mentorship Program and the driving force behind the success of Family Faith Nights, James's contemplation of the spiritual aspect of his leadership and community service is critical. Although the tangible achievements of these endeavors were evident, James recognized that their true essence resided in a more profound, introspective realm. It was imperative to refocus the community's attention on this spiritual core and reaffirm the source of their strength for themselves and others.

The question that lingered in James's mind and that he knew was silently echoed in the hearts of many was, "Where is God through all of this?" It was a question of faith, of seeing the invisible hand at work, not just in the good times but especially through the trials and the everyday efforts to uplift one another. He shared his struggles and the silent echoes with his pastor and some elders in his faith. Pastor Alinko acknowledged that through some of his conversations and counseling in the community, James was not alone in this silent spiritual struggle.

To address this, Pastor Alinko organized a unique "In the Footsteps of Faith" retreat to renew and deepen the community's spiritual connections. The retreat would be held over a weekend at a peaceful lakeside camp nearby. In this place, the beauty of nature would remind everyone of the divine presence in the world around them.

The retreat included prayer and meditation sessions, sacred discussions by various faith leaders, and personal testimony sharing. This sacred session allowed participants to reflect and share where they encounter God in their lives and the community efforts. It was an opportunity for introspection, to acknowledge the unseen guidance and support that had bolstered their initiatives.

One of the most powerful moments came during a session called 'Seeing the Unseen,' where community members were invited to share personal stories of faith during difficult times. These stories were about overcoming challenges, personal growth, and transformation, inspiring hope and resilience in everyone present.

In his turn, James shared his journey, from military service to the recent challenges in Alaska and his leadership in Fort Reachie. "In each chapter of my life, in every challenge we have faced together as a community, I see the workings of a greater plan," James reflected. "Grand gestures do not always mark God's presence, but often in the quiet moments, we find strength during trials and in the joy of serving others." This retreat has deepened the community's spiritual connections and transformed my leadership, infusing it with a renewed sense of divine purpose.

The retreat also featured workshops on consciously incorporating faith into daily life and community service. Participants united in their pursuit of spiritual growth. They felt a renewed sense of purpose and spiritual connection as the retreat drew close with a serene sunset service by the lake. They sang hymns that echoed across the water, their voices a testament to their revitalized faith and unity, a shared commitment to making a difference in their community.

Returning from the retreat, the community of Fort Reachie felt more cohesive and spiritually charged. These initiatives were now imbued with a renewed sense of divine purpose, enriching the practical aspects of community service with a more profound spiritual commitment. James documented this spiritual renewal in his ongoing journal, noting, "This weekend, we walked in the footsteps of our faith, and in doing so, we remembered that God walks with us in every endeavor, every act of kindness, and every challenge.

This unseen strength binds all our efforts and ensures that even in moments of doubt, we are never truly alone." As Fort Reachie moved forward, the balance between faith, family, and service became more pronounced, driving the community to new heights of compassion and cooperation, all underpinned by a profound acknowledgment of their spiritual foundations.

In the weeks after the retreat, James observed a noticeable change in the Fort Reachie community. A plunging sense of tranquility appeared to flow through their interactions and events. It was as if the retreat had not only refreshed their spirits but had also woven a thread of calm assurance through the heart of the town. This change inspired James to continue exploring ways to integrate these spiritual insights into daily life and community actions even further.

To harness the energy from the retreat, James convinces the community elders and leaders to initiate a volunteering opportunity called 'Faith in Action Days,' where the community would actively apply their faith through service projects around town. These were not just opportunities to help; they were opportunities for the practical applications of their spiritual beliefs, a way to live out the teachings they embraced during their time of reflection.

Each project began with a prayer by different community members, highlighting the focus on inclusivity and the shared spiritual mission. Whether restoring a family's home, planting a community garden, or organizing a day of activities and companionship at the local senior center, each activity was charged with a purpose that transcended the mere act of service. These were opportunities to help and for practical applications of their spiritual beliefs. It was a way to live out the teachings they embraced during their time of reflection. This practical aspect of faith in action empowered the participants, making them feel capable of making a tangible difference in their community.

One particularly inspiring project was the renovation of an old playground. The space had fallen into disrepair, and many children in the town had stopped visiting it. The community decided it was the perfect opportunity for a Faith in Action Day. Volunteers of all ages came together, their efforts fueled by a sermon about the joy and innocence of children and how creating safe and joyful spaces for them was a reflection of divine care. As they painted, repaired, and cleaned, the volunteers shared stories of their childhoods, their voices mingling with laughter and the rhythmic strokes of paintbrushes. The project's completion led to restoring the playground to its original condition.

The community united to mark the reopening with a lively neighborhood picnic.

They shared prayers and watched as children reveled in the renewed space, demonstrating the community's unwavering faith in action. Seeing the impact of these projects, James decided to compile these stories and reflections into a book titled "Faith in Action: The Fort Reachie Experience."

This book will serve as a definitive guide for other communities. It will provide a blueprint for integrating faith into community service. It will also help demonstrate that one can actively live out their spiritual beliefs to effect real-world change.

The book was filled with personal anecdotes, photos of the projects, and templates for organizing similar initiatives. It also included sections on the theological underpinnings that supported these activities, written in collaboration with local clergies. When published, the book received attention far beyond Fort Reachie, inspiring other towns to adopt similar programs. Through these ongoing efforts, James helped to create a legacy of active faith in Fort Reachie that inspired his community and others to look beyond themselves to see their spiritual beliefs as a catalyst for tangible, positive change in the world. The community had shown that when faith moves from being a personal belief to a community action, it can transform not just individual lives but the very fabric of society.

CHAPTER 13

LEGACY OF LIGHT

At the end of the year, Fort Reachie underwent a remarkable transformation beyond just being blanketed by winter's snow. Thanks to COL James Aish's guidance, the community has become an inspiration and a prime example of positive change driven by the community. This incredible shift was brought about by shared values and faith, leading to concrete accomplishments. The accomplishments, to mention a few, are establishing a community garden to provide fresh produce and revamping the local park into a safe and welcoming space for children. It also includes instituting a mentorship program to foster the growth of young leaders.

James sat in his office at the community center, surrounded by photographs of the various projects and people that had defined his recent years. Each image told a story of collaboration, resilience, and faith in action. They were all visual testaments to the profound impact of his and the community's efforts. His eyes lingered on a picture taken during the first Family Faith Night, a reminder of where this all began. At that moment, a sense of distinction and accomplishment washed over him, evidence of the power of community-driven change.

As he reflected on the journey, James decided it was time to compile these experiences and lessons into a comprehensive narrative. Documenting the history of Fort Reachie's transformation required much more effort than anticipated. It was a meticulous process of selecting the most impactful stories, distilling the key lessons, and weaving them into a coherent narrative. The result was a blueprint for others to follow, a book titled *Legacy of Light*, aiming to illuminate the path for communities worldwide to harness the power of faith and collective action.

In preparing his manuscript, James and Elizabeth contacted community members to contribute their stories. They wanted the book to have diverse voices like the young mother who found strength in the community to overcome personal trials, the veteran who rediscovered his purpose through service, and the teenagers who grew into leaders through the mentorship program.

Each story would weave into the next, creating a rich tapestry of life and change. As *Legacy of Light* came together, James and Elizabeth organized a series of community gatherings to read excerpts, discuss content, and gather feedback. These gatherings served as editorial sessions and celebrations of the community's achievements. They were held in various locations around town, from the newly renovated park to the expanded community garden, each site a backdrop to the stories shared.

James introduced a new initiative during one such gathering: the Lightkeepers program. This program aims to sustain and expand the revitalizing principles of Fort Reachie. Lightkeepers would be trained community leaders responsible for initiating projects, resolving conflicts, and fostering spiritual growth within the community. They would ensure that the legacy of Fort Reachie would continue, even as the original participants aged or moved on. This program was designed for everyone in the community, emphasizing each member's integral role in shaping the community's future.

The villagers embraced the announcement enthusiastically, and many young adults eagerly signed up, inspired by the chance to contribute and lead. James felt deeply satisfied knowing he was leaving behind a physical, doctrinal legacy and a living, breathing one. He is leaving behind a village equipped to thrive and inspire. *Legacy of Light* was published in the spring, its release timed with a town-wide celebration that mirrored the communal spirit of the book. Copies were sent to libraries, schools, and community centers; James even arranged for copies to be distributed at a national community leadership conference.

As James watched the community come together to celebrate the launch, he knew his role had shifted. He was no longer just a leader but a steward of a vision that had grown beyond him. He saw his reflections in the young faces around him, in the eager discussions about projects and dreams, and he knew that Fort Reachie was in capable hands.

The book's final chapter was intentionally blank and titled "Your Chapter." This chapter, which was to be written by the community, was an invitation for others to pick up on where this story had ended. It was for the citizens to continue the work of building community, faith, and hope. This book initiative was more than just a call to action. It was more of recognizing the community's power and responsibility in shaping its future.

Sitting quietly at the back during the celebration, James and Elizabeth held hands with both faces filled with smiles as they watched the festivities. The laughter, the planning, and the shared stories of trials and triumphs create a beautiful echo of the journey. Fort Reachie has taught their family that every community has the potential to illuminate the darkest times, turn challenges into victories, and forge a legacy that shines brightly. This chapter guides the way forward for all willing to lead with faith, serve with love, and live purposefully.

CHAPTER 14

THE LIFELINE OF CONNECTION

Years later, COL James Aish, a compassionate member of the military community, took some time in his study during the onset of winter to reflect. He reflected on an important issue that had deeply impacted many lives, including his own. He pondered the unique challenges of military life, such as stress, demands, and the potential for isolation. These reflections inspired the final chapter of his new book, which emphasizes the crucial message about the importance of relationships, connections, and support in preventing suicide.

The book's last chapter, "Connect to Protect: Support is Within Reach," sheds light on the common yet often overlooked struggles soldiers and their families face. This chapter discusses silent struggles like long separations, the anxiety of deployments, and the internal battles that remained long after the physical ones had ended. James shares stories, some anonymized, about individuals who have grappled with their darkest moments while feeling disconnected from their support networks.

He wrote that maintaining solid personal connections is essential. "In the military," James penned, "we are trained to be tough, to withstand physical and psychological pressures. But our bonds with each other, our friends, families, and even superiors, truly fortify our spirits against the trials we face." James highlighted how critical it was for families and friends to understand their role in the mental well-being of their loved ones in the service. "It is not merely about being present," he noted. "It is about being proactive, reaching out, and ensuring that the lines of communication are always open. It is about ensuring no one feels they must suffer in silence or go through it alone."

To provide practical advice, James discussed the array of support systems available within the military community. He listed resources like the Department of Behavioral Health, which offers counseling and therapy services, chaplains who provide spiritual support, the Military Family Life counselor who assists with family-related issues, and Army Community Services, which included the Employee Assistance Program within the Army Substance Abuse Program that offers confidential counseling and referral services. James stressed the importance of recognizing when someone might need help and how to offer that help effectively. Sometimes, he noted, it was as simple as lending an ear or starting a conversation.

Addressing lethal means safety, James included a segment on the preventive measures to control access to potentially harmful items. "While having access to lethal means does not make everyone a risk," he wrote, "for someone in crisis, easy access could pose a higher threat. It is about preventive measures, about reducing risks wherever possible." In closing, James sought to inspire a sense of collective responsibility.

He urged every reader, especially those within military communities, to see themselves as part of a broader support network. "We have a moral duty to protect each other," he asserted. "To watch, to listen, and to act. If you sense someone is at risk, do not hesitate. Reach out, offer help, and make that call. Your action could save a life."

He concluded the chapter with a call to arms for compassion and vigilance, reminding everyone that while military life might be fraught with challenges, the community's strength, resilience, and unwavering support for each member are its pillars. "Let this book serve as a reminder to all of us," James wrote, "of the power we hold to change lives. In Fort Reachie, "Let us Connect to create a community where everyone is supported and valued, and no one is ever alone."

With that, James set down his pen, hoping his words would resonate, educate, and perhaps most importantly, catalyze action that could turn the tide for those struggling in silence. As he leaned back in his chair, he felt a deep, enduring hope that his efforts would help light the path for many to find their way back from the brink.

CHAPTER 15

ECHOES OF CHANGE

Under COL James Aish's stewardship, Fort Reachie's community underwent a remarkable transformation as the seasons changed. The success of the 'Faith in Action Days' and the publication of *Faith in Action: The Fort Reachie Experience* piqued interest beyond the town's borders. It led to tangible changes within the community playgrounds, gardens, and renovated homes. However, the profound sense of unity and purpose that the residents displayed was a testament that truly captured James's attention and his leadership.

With the increasing recognition of their community efforts, Fort Reachie found itself at the center of a growing movement. Inspired by James's leadership, other communities began reaching out, seeking guidance on how they, too, could integrate faith and service meaningfully. In response, the local leaders set up an outreach initiative to guide other towns through establishing their Faith in Action Days.

The initiative started with a symposium in Fort Reachie. James and other community leaders shared their experiences, strategies, and outcomes on this platform. The event drew a diverse audience like clergies, community organizers, local politicians, and educators. They were all eager to learn and be inspired to replicate the town's success in their communities. During the symposium, Pastor Alinko, through the help of James's wife and other local leaders, seized the opportunity to introduce a workshop titled "Building Community through Faith," This workshop will combine theoretical teachings with practical, hands-on sessions where participants could plan real projects to implement in their communities. The workshop emphasized the importance of inclusivity, ensuring that initiatives welcomed all community members, regardless of their faith backgrounds, to participate in shaping their environment.

Mrs. Elizabeth Aish led one of the most impactful sessions. Apart from being James' wife, Elizabeth has worked alongside James in both his civilian and military endeavors as a trauma and crisis licensed counselor. She honed her expertise in community engagement through her work with the Family Faith Nights. Elizabeth shared a powerful insight about the transformative power of listening to a community's needs and hopes. "Transformation begins when we open our hearts and ears," she explained. "It's about more than just addressing physical needs; it is about understanding the emotional and spiritual aspirations of the people we serve." This perspective resonated deeply with the audience, reinforcing the importance of empathy and understanding in community initiatives.

The symposium culminated in a community service project right in Fort Reachie. All participants gathered to participate in a large-scale restoration of the local community center. The project allowed them to put into practice the principles they had discussed and gave them a tangible sense of the impact such efforts could have. The symposium's success paved the way for an online forum. Communities could continue exchanging ideas, successes, challenges, and resources in this virtual space.

Elizabeth played an active role in the forum, providing advice and encouragement and occasionally organizing virtual meetups and physical talks over coffee, especially for young mothers. This platform served as a beacon of ongoing connection and mutual support among the growing network of faith-based service communities.

As winter approached, bringing the reflective quiet of snow-covered landscapes, James took a moment to pen his thoughts in a new chapter of his ongoing journal. He wrote about the expansion of Fort Reachie's influence, not as a self-congratulatory note but as an affidavit to what faith, combined with action, could achieve. "This is not just about what we have built or fixed," James wrote. "It is about the bridges we have built between hearts and across communities. Each project and each initiative strengthen not only the physical infrastructures of our towns but also the spiritual and emotional bonds that tie us together. We are crafting a legacy of empathy, action, and hope as a beacon for those who believe in the power of community and faith to change the world."

James and Elizabeth found a deeply felt sense of peace in the quiet snowfall outside their window. Despite the ongoing work that awaited them, they took comfort in simply watching the snowflakes gently descend, each one a gentle reminder of change. As they sipped their coffee, holding hands, they appreciated the serene moment, feeling thankful for each other's company.

CHAPTER 16

EPILOGUE

For those facing the difficult journey of mental health challenges, this book is more than just a story of community and faith. It stands as a symbol of resilience, optimism, and personalized support for you. It recognizes that your battles may often go unnoticed by the world and acknowledges the relentless inner turmoil you endure. While the tales of unity and collective strength in Fort Reachie may feel distant from your personal or silent struggles, their message may sincerely resonate with your journey.

This book offers practical strategies for dealing with mental health challenges, including seeking help, using community resources, and sharing your story. The core truth that illuminates every page of this story is this: You do not have to walk your path alone. Just as Fort Reachie extended its hands in times of need, support systems are ready to embrace you. Reaching out for help, engaging with community resources, or simply sharing your story can be the first brave step toward recovery.

You are not alone in your fight. Your community, whether it is your neighborhood, online support groups, or mental health centers, is a taproot you can rely on. Additionally, let this book remind you that your journey through mental health challenges does not define you—it refines you. Like the citizens of Fort Reachie, who transformed trials into triumphs, your struggles can forge strength and empathy, qualities that the world dearly needs.

Like James, you have the potential to turn your deepest trials into testimonies of survival and hope, which can, in turn, reinforce your resilience and inner strength. In "Legacy of Light," we saw individuals who overcame their shadows together through the power of shared stories and collective action. Your story, too, is valuable and deserves to be heard. In sharing it, you find healing and light the way for others who might still be searching in the dark.

We all possess the potential to be a force of comfort and safety for one another. You can become a beacon of hope, like Fort Reachie, inspiring others with your resilience and courage. Your voice matters, and your story can make a difference. Furthermore, remember, like the open pages in the Legacy of Light's final chapter, your story is ongoing. Each day is a new opportunity to write a narrative of recovery and hope. Your experiences, struggles, and victories add depth to the broader human story, contributing bravery, perseverance, and compassion lessons.

So, to those feeling weighed down by mental health struggles, take heart. Continue to fight, continue to hope, and continue to connect with those around you. For some of us who may find ourselves in a place like Fort reachie, remember that you can also be the one to light the path for others. The path to healing is often walked in steps, not leaps. Moreover, with each small step, know that a community of hearts and hands, seen and unseen, walks with you.

It takes courage to fill the pages of your life with a story of hope, but in doing so, you can inspire yourself and others. If you want to learn more about weaving a tale of hope, consider checking out my new book, "The Silent Chapter: Healing and Overcoming Your Silent Struggles." Just like the community of Fort Reachie, I hope you find strength and guidance through unity, support, and shared understanding.

FROM MY HEART

Dear Warriors and Family Members,

It has been an honor to serve as a chaplain. This role has allowed me to witness the profound strength and resilience of our military personnel and their families. As we close the pages of this book, I want to address you directly and remind you of the many ways military life can affect us physically, spiritually, mentally, and emotionally.

The journey of soldiers and their families involves exceptional sacrifice, and the stresses that come with this service can sometimes feel overwhelming. Knowing that you are not alone on this path and that help is available to guide you through it is critical. I want to assure you on behalf of all military chaplains that we are always here for you, providing unwavering support.

We are trained to offer spiritual guidance, emotional support, and a listening ear. Please do not hesitate to ask whether you need counsel, a prayer, or talk to someone. Remember the proverb: "Where no counsel is, the people fall: but in the multitude of counselors there is safety" (Proverbs 11:14). We are here to support you and pray with you in every way possible.

This book, a compilation of stories and lessons from the heart of Fort Reachie, is a testament to the power of community and connection. Let it serve as a reminder to all of us of the crucial role we play in each other's lives. We have a moral duty to protect and support our service members and their families now more than ever. The bonds we forge, the support we offer, and the vigilance we maintain can be life-saving.

If you are concerned for someone's safety or if they are at an imminent risk for suicide, I urge you not to leave them alone. Immediate action can make all the difference. You can contact the National Suicide Prevention

Lifeline, available 24/7, at **988**. Alternatively, reach out to a chaplain (military chaplains offer 100% confidentiality), visit any behavioral health center, consult a healthcare provider, or, in urgent cases, go to an emergency room or dial **911** in the USA.

Our commitment to each other's well-being strengthens us as a force, community, and nation. Let us uphold this honor and sacred duty to watch over one another with care and compassion, ensuring that no one faces their darkest moments alone.

Remember that your chaplains, leaders, and community are ever-present as we part ways through these written words. Reach out and find the support that can help you through this. Together, as we commit to defending our nation, we stand firm against the tides of challenges, united in our mission to protect and uplift each other.

With the most profound respect and unwavering support,

Remain blessed & inspired!
Dr. Aigbefo D. Ehihi
Chaplain, United States Army.

ABOUT THE AUTHOR

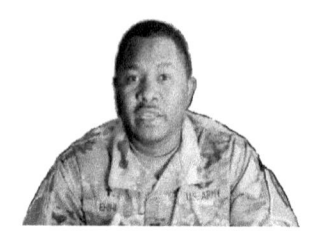

Dr. Aigbefo D. Ehihi is a distinguished coach, pastor, and military chaplain, revered for his unwavering dedication to ministry and military service. His extensive background in theology, leadership, and social and behavioral sciences equips him with remarkable expertise. Dr. Ehihi passionately engages in various outreach initiatives alongside his family, translating his calling into impactful deeds. He is also the esteemed author of the bestselling books "So Many Friends, So Little Friendship" and "Living Every Day With The Cross," which have furnished countless listeners and readers with inspired and uplifting messages.

ABOUT THE BOOK

In "**Hold Fast: A Story of Hope & Intervention**," retired Colonel James Aish reveals how the power of community and faith can transform lives, especially among military families grappling with the unseen wounds of service. The book shares personal stories, practical strategies, and expert advice on coping with mental health challenges and suicide prevention. Returning to his hometown, Fort Reachie, James ignites a movement of resilience and support, proving that no soldier or family should ever battle alone. This compelling narrative not only offers practical strategies for suicide prevention but also inspires readers to connect, support, and protect each other in a world where hope and help are always within reach but merely utilized. Join James and me in "**Hold Fast: A Story of Hope & Intervention**," and discover how you can strengthen the bonds of community and faith to make a lasting impact in the lives of military families and beyond.

OTHER BOOKS BY DR. EHIHI

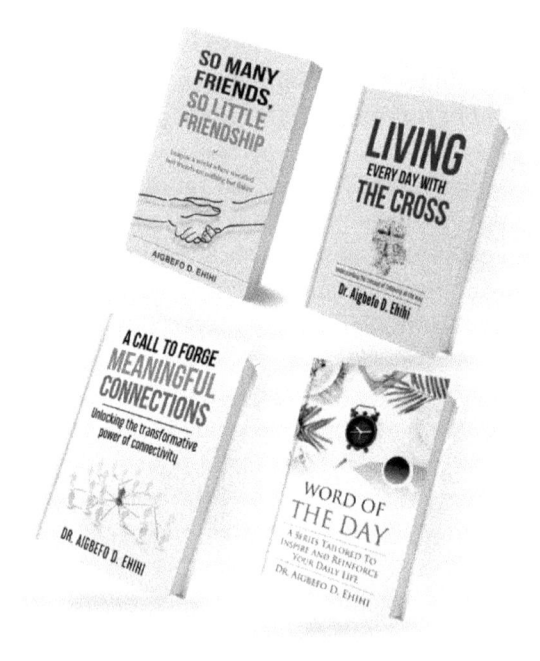

Available in any major bookstore(s)

NOTES

Milton Keynes UK
Ingram Content Group UK Ltd.
UKHW030348240824
447344UK00001BA/2